Amazing Diabetic recipes for everyone

50 amazing recipes to enjoy every day

Roseann Smith

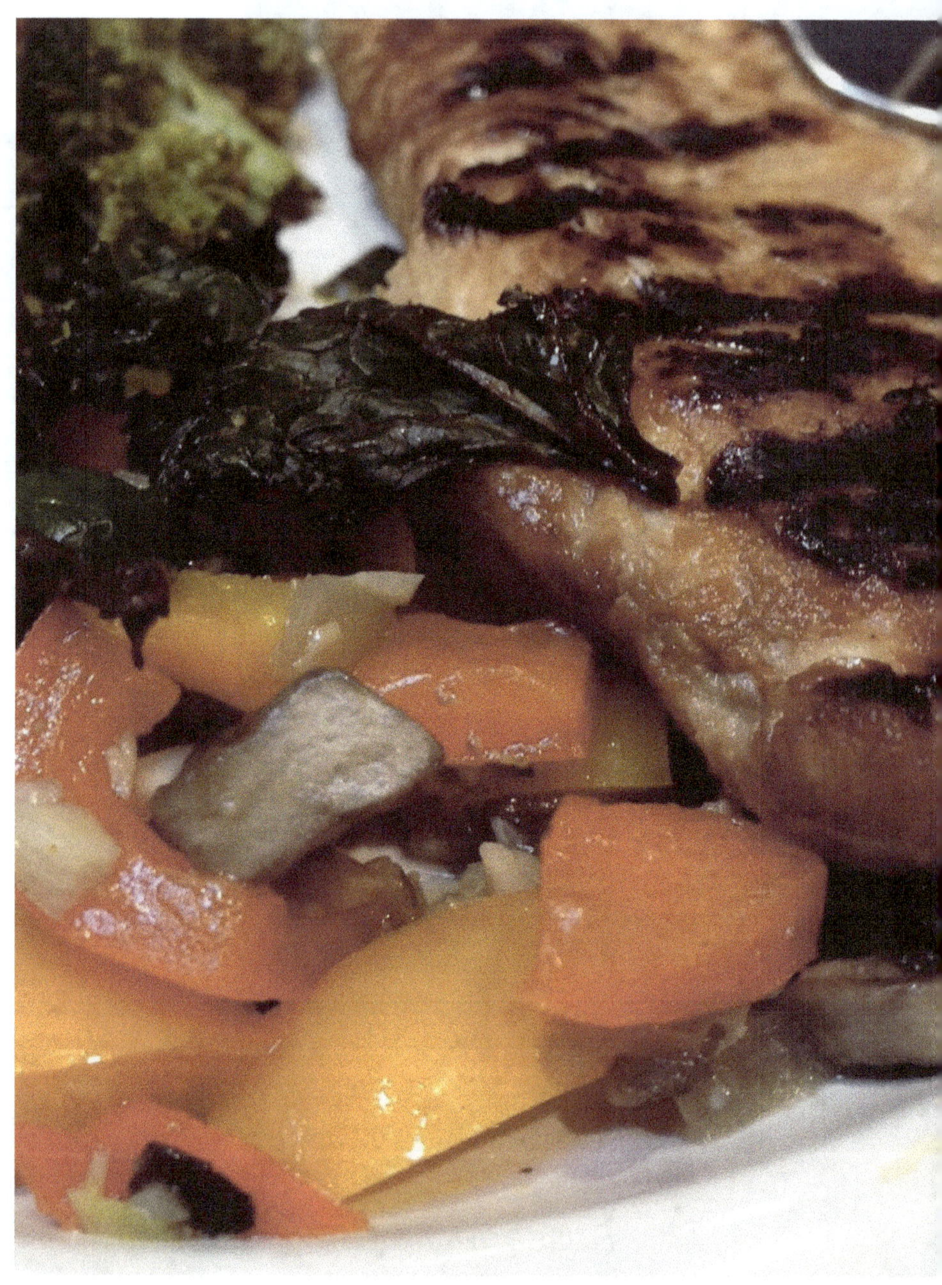

Disclaimer Notice:

Please note the information contained within this document is for educational and entertainment purposes only. All effort has been executed to present accurate, up to date, and reliable, complete information. No warranties of any kind are declared or implied. Readers acknowledge that the author is not engaging in the rendering of legal, financial, medical or professional advice. The content within this book has been derived from various sources. Please consult a licensed professional before attempting any techniques outlined in this book. By reading this document, the reader agrees that under no circumstances is the author responsible for any losses, direct or indirect, which are incurred as a result of the use of information contained within this document, including, but not limited to, — errors, omissions, or inaccuracies.

Table of Contents

Pea And Mint Soup 7

Kale & Tofu Salad 9

Tofu With Brussels Sprouts 12

Grains Combo 15

Mixed Veggie Salad 17

Zucchini With Tomatoes 20

Tofu With Brussels Sprout 23

Baked Veggies Combo 26

Lentils Chili 28

Fried Tofu Hotpot 32

Seitan Curry 33

Split Pea Stew 34

Grilled Potatoes In A Packet 35

Seitan Roast 37

Eggplant Curry 38

Irish Stew 39

Vegetarian Split Pea Soup In A Crock Pot 40

Thai Peanut, Carrot, & Shrimp Soup 42

Ham Asparagus Soup 45

Cabbage Soup 49

Chickpea Soup 50

Meatball Stew 51

Squash Soup 53

French Onion Soup 55

Cherry Stew 56

Curried Carrot Soup 57

Vegan Cream Soup With Avocado & Zucchini 59

Kebab Stew 61

Meatless Ball Soup 62

Tofu Soup 64

Chicken Zoodle Soup 67

Cheese Cream Soup With Chicken & Cilantro 68

Spicy Pepper Soup 70

Awesome Chicken Enchilada Soup 71

Zucchini-basil Soup 73

Sweet And Sour Soup 75

Curried Shrimp & Green Bean Soup 76

Beef Borscht Soup 78

Broccoli & Spinach Soup 80

Vegetable Chicken Soup 82

Beef Barley Soup.. 84

Sirloin Carrot Soup 87

Mexican Chicken Soup 89

Mushroom Cream Soup With Herbs 91

Beef & Mushroom Barley Soup 93

Spicy Chicken Pepper Stew.. 96

Cream Pepper Stew.. 98

Easy Beef Mushroom Stew 101

Summer Squash Soup With Crispy Chickpeas 103

Healthy Chicken Kale Soup 106

Pea And Mint Soup

Servings: 2

Cooking Time: 35 Minutes

Ingredients:

- 1lb green peas
- 2 cups low sodium vegetable broth
- 3tbsp mint sauce

Directions:

1. Mix all the ingredients in your Instant Pot.
2. Cook on Stew for 35 minutes.
3. Release the pressure naturally.
4. Blend into a rough soup.

Nutrition Info: Calories: 130 Carbs: 17 Sugar: 4 Fat: 5 Protein: 19 GL: 11

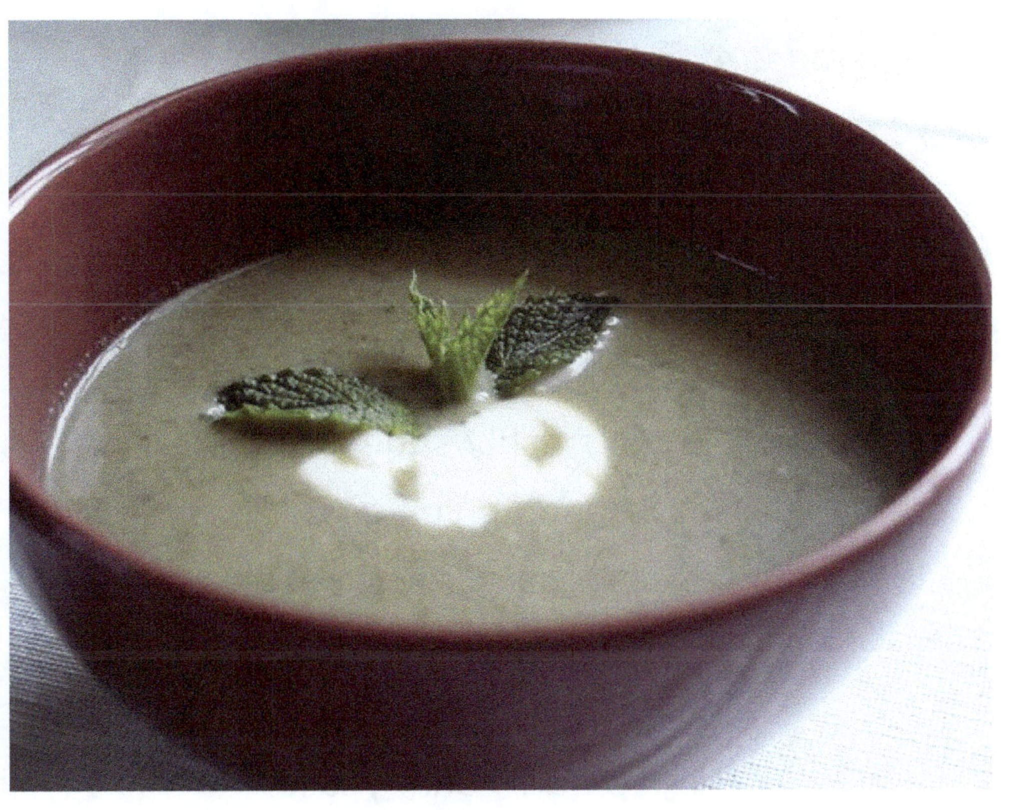

Kale & Tofu Salad

Servings: 4

Cooking Time: 15 Minutes

Ingredients:

- 1 block tofu, sliced into cubes
- ¼ cup Worcestershire sauce
- ¼ cup freshly squeezed lemon juice
- 1 teaspoon onion powder
- 1 teaspoon garlic powder
- 3 teaspoons olive oil
- 8 cups kale, chopped
- ¼ cup nutritional yeast
- ¼ cup pumpkin seeds, toasted
- ½ cup Caesar dressing
- 1 avocado, sliced

Directions:

1. Dry the tofu with paper towel.
2. In a bowl, mix the Worcestershire sauce, lemon juice, onion powder and garlic powder.
3. Coat the tofu with this mixture.
4. Let it stand for 15 minutes.
5. Discard the marinade.
6. Pour the oil in a pan over medium heat.
7. Cook the tofu until golden brown on all sides.
8. Drain the oil and set aside.
9. In a bowl, toss the kale in nutritional yeast.
10. Divide into containers.
11. Top each container with croutons and pumpkin seeds.
12. Pour dressing on top and serve with avocado slices.

Nutrition Info: Calories 400 Total Fat 28 g
Saturated Fat 4 g Cholesterol 6 mg Sodium 423
mg Total Carbohydrate 19 g Dietary Fiber 9 g
Total Sugars 2 g Protein 20 g Potassium 670
mg

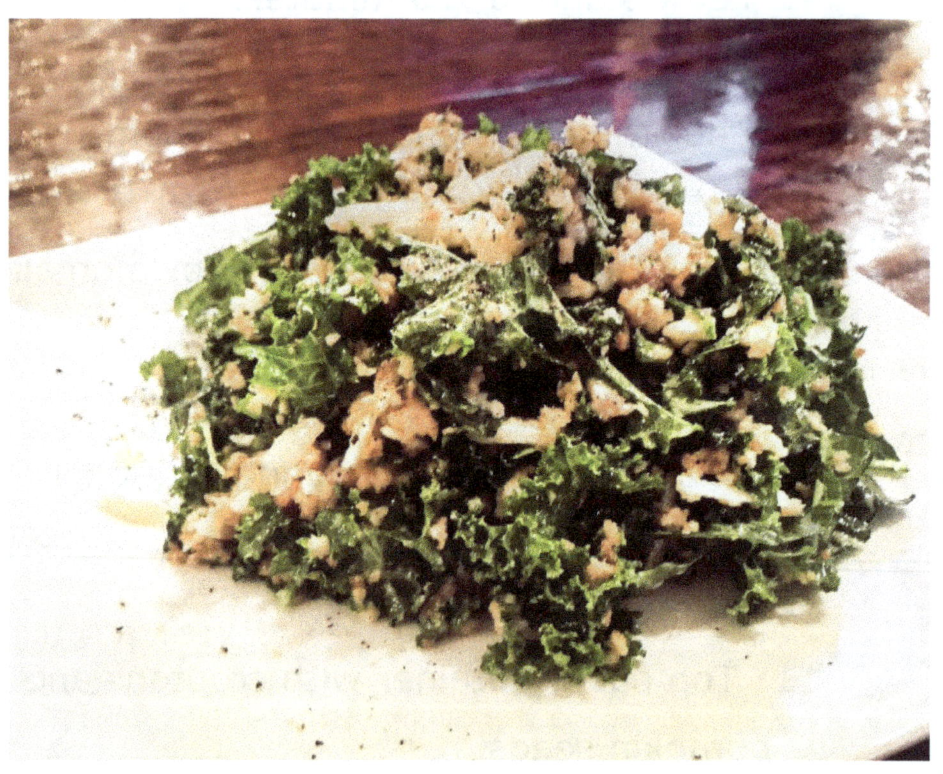

Tofu With Brussels Sprouts

Servings: 3

Cooking Time: 15 Minutes

Ingredients:

- 1½ tablespoons olive oil, divided
- 8 ounces' extra-firm tofu, drained, pressed, and cut into slices
- 2 garlic cloves, chopped
- 1/3 cup pecans, toasted, and chopped
- 1 tablespoon unsweetened applesauce
- ¼ cup fresh cilantro, chopped
- ½ pound Brussels sprouts, trimmed and cut into wide ribbons
- ¾ pound mixed bell peppers, seeded and sliced

Directions:

1. In a skillet, heat ½ tablespoon of the oil over medium heat and sauté the tofu and for about 6–7 minutes, or until golden-brown.
2. Add the garlic and pecans and sauté for about 1 minute.
3. Add the applesauce and cook for about 2 minutes.
4. Stir in the cilantro and remove from heat.
5. Transfer tofu into a plate and set aside
6. In the same skillet, heat the remaining oil over medium-high heat and cook the Brussels sprouts and bell peppers for about 5 minutes.
7. Stir in the tofu and remove from the heat.
8. Serve immediately.

Nutrition Info: Calories 238 Total Fat 17.8 g Saturated Fat 2 g Cholesterol 0 mg Sodium 26 mg Total Carbs 13.6 g Fiber 4.8 g Sugar 4.5 g Protein 11.8 g

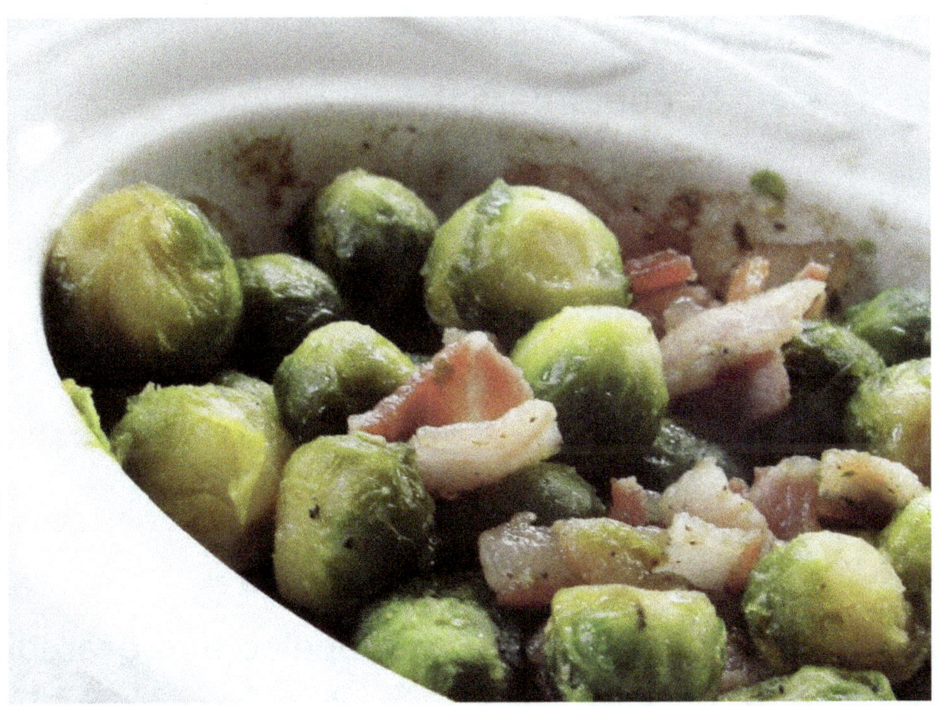

Grains Combo

Servings: 6

Cooking Time: 35 Minutes

Ingredients:

- ¾ cup amaranth
- 1 cup quinoa, rinsed
- ¼ cup wild rice
- 4¼ cups filtered water
- 2 teaspoons ground cumin
- ½ teaspoon paprika
- Salt, as required
- 1¼ cups boiled chickpeas
- 2 medium carrots, peeled and grated
- 1 garlic clove, minced
- Ground black pepper, as required

Directions:

1. In a large pan, add the amaranth, quinoa, wild rice, water and spices over medium-high heat and bring to a boil.

2. Now, reduce the heat to medium-low and simmer, covered for about 20-25 minutes.

3. Stir in remaining ingredients and simmer for about 3-5 minutes.

4. Serve hot.

5. Meal Prep Tip: Transfer the grains mixture into a large bowl and set aside to cool. Divide the mixture into 6 containers evenly. Cover the containers and refrigerate for 1 day. Reheat in the microwave before serving.

Nutrition Info: Calories 365 Total Fat 5.6 g Saturated Fat 0.6 g Cholesterol 0 mg Total Carbs 64 g Sugar 5.8 g Fiber 12 g Sodium 58 mg Potassium 686 mg Protein 16.4 g

Mixed Veggie Salad

Servings: 8

Ingredients:

- For Dressing:
- 1/3 cup olive oil
- ½ cup fresh lemon juice
- 1 tablespoon fresh ginger, grated
- 2 teaspoons mustard
- 4-6 drops liquid stevia
- ¼ teaspoon salt
- For Salad:
- 2 avocados, peeled, pitted and chopped
- 2 tablespoons fresh lemon juice
- 2 cups fresh baby spinach, torn
- 2 cups small broccoli florets
- 1 cup red cabbage, shredded
- 1 cup purple cabbage, shredded
- 2 large carrots, peeled and grated

- 1 small orange bell pepper, seeded and sliced into matchsticks
- 1 small yellow bell pepper, seeded and sliced into matchsticks
- ½ cup fresh parsley leaves, chopped
- 1 cup walnuts, chopped

Directions:

1. For dressing: in a food processor, add all ingredients and pulse until well combined.
2. In a large bowl, add the avocado slices and drizzle with lemon juice.
3. Add the remaining vegetables and mix.
4. Place the dressing and toss to coat well.
5. Serve immediately.
6. Meal Prep Tip: Transfer dressing into a small jar and refrigerate for 1 day. In 8 containers, divide avocado and remaining vegetables. Refrigerate for 1

day. Before serving, drizzle each
portion with dressing and serve.

Nutrition Info: Calories 314 Total Fat 28.1 g
Saturated Fat 4 g Cholesterol 0 mg Total Carbs
14.1 g Sugar 4.3g Fiber 6.9 g Sodium 113 mg
Potassium 642 mg Protein 6.8 g

Zucchini With Tomatoes

Servings: 8

Cooking Time: 11 Minutes

Ingredients:

- 6 medium zucchinis, chopped roughly
- 1-pound cherry tomatoes
- 2 small onions, chopped roughly
- 2 tablespoons fresh basil, chopped
- 1 cup water
- 1 tablespoon olive oil
- 2 garlic cloves, minced
- Salt and ground black pepper, as required

Directions:

1. In the Instant Pot, place oil and press "Sauté". Now add the onion, garlic, ginger, and spices and cook for about 3-4 minutes.
2. Add the zucchinis and tomatoes and cook for about 1-2 minutes.
3. Press "Cancel" and stir in the remaining ingredients except basil.
4. Close the lid and place the pressure valve to "Seal" position.
5. Press "Manual" and cook under "High Pressure" for about 5 minutes.
6. Press "Cancel" and allow a "Natural" release.
7. Open the lid and transfer the vegetable mixture onto a serving platter.
8. Garnish with basil and serve.

Nutrition Info: Calories: 57 Fats: 2.1g Carbohydrates: 9gSugar: 4.8gProteins: 2.5g Sodium: 39mg

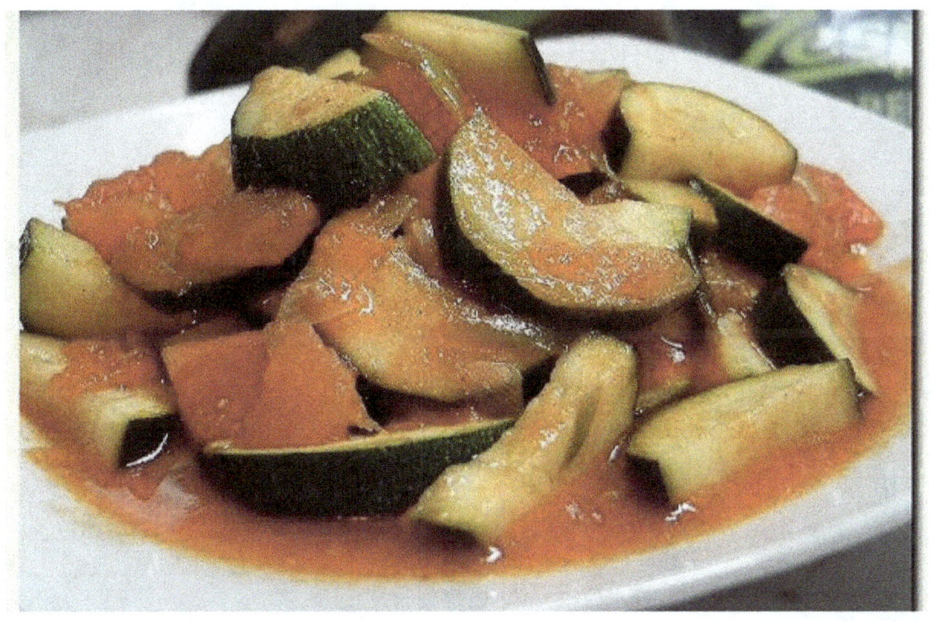

Tofu With Brussels Sprout

Servings: 4

Cooking Time: 15 Minutes

Ingredients:

- 1 tablespoon olive oil, divided
- 8 ounces extra-firm tofu, drained, pressed and cut into slices
- 2 garlic cloves, chopped
- 1/3 cup pecans, toasted and chopped
- 1 tablespoon unsweetened applesauce
- ¼ cup fresh cilantro, chopped
- ¾ pound Brussels sprouts, trimmed and cut into wide ribbons

Directions:

1. In a skillet, heat ½ tablespoon of the oil over medium heat and sauté the tofu and for about 6-7 minutes or until golden brown.

2. Add the garlic and pecans and sauté for about 1 minute.

3. Add the applesauce and cook for about 2 minutes.

4. Stir in the cilantro and remove from heat.

5. Transfer tofu into a plate and set aside

6. In the same skillet, heat the remaining oil over medium-high heat and cook the Brussels sprouts for about 5 minutes.

7. Stir in the tofu and remove from the heat.

8. Serve immediately.

9. Meal Prep Tip: Remove the tofu mixture from heat and set aside to cool completely. In 4 containers, divide the

tofu mixture evenly and refrigerate for about 2 days. Reheat in microwave before serving.

Nutrition Info: Calories 204 Total Fat 15.5 g Saturated Fat 1.8 g Cholesterol 0 mg Total Carbs 11.5 g Sugar 3 g Fiber 4.8 g Sodium 27 mg Potassium 468 mg Protein 9.9 g

Baked Veggies Combo

Servings: 8

Cooking Time: 40 Minutes

Ingredients:

- 2 large zucchinis, sliced
- 1 large yellow squash, sliced
- 3 cups fresh broccoli florets
- 1 pound fresh asparagus, trimmed
- 2 garlic cloves, minced
- 1 tablespoon fresh rosemary, minced
- 1 tablespoon fresh thyme, minced
- ½ teaspoon ground cumin
- ½ teaspoon red pepper flakes, crushed
- ¼ teaspoon cayenne pepper
- 2 tablespoons olive oil
- Salt, as required

Directions:

1. Preheat the oven to 400 degrees F. Line 2 large baking sheets with aluminum foil.

2. In a large bowl, add all ingredients and toss to coat well.

3. Divide the vegetables mixture onto prepared baking sheets and spread in a single layer.

4. Roast for about 35-40 minutes.

5. Remove from oven and serve.

6. Meal Prep Tip: Remove from oven and set the veggies aside to cool completely. Transfer the veggie mixture into 8 containers and refrigerate for 2-3 days. Reheat in microwave before serving.

Nutrition Info: Calories 77 Total Fat 4 g Saturated Fat 0.6 g Cholesterol 0 mg Total Carbs 9.4 g Sugar 3.8 g Fiber 3.8 g Sodium 45 mg Potassium 554 mg Protein 3.8 g

Lentils Chili

Servings: 8

Cooking Time: 2 Hours 20 Minutes

Ingredients:

- 2 teaspoons olive oil
- 1 large onion, chopped
- 3 medium carrot, peeled and chopped
- 4 celery stalks, chopped
- 2 garlic cloves, minced
- 1 jalapeño pepper, seeded and chopped
- ½ tablespoon dried thyme, crushed
- 1 tablespoon chipotle chili powder
- ½ tablespoon cayenne pepper
- 1½ tablespoons ground coriander
- 1½ tablespoons ground cumin
- 1 teaspoon ground turmeric

- Ground black pepper, as required
- 1 tomato, chopped finely
- 1 pound lentils, rinsed
- 8 cups low-sodium vegetable broth
- 6 cups fresh spinach
- ½ cup fresh cilantro, chopped

Directions:

1. In a large pan, heat the oil over medium heat and sauté the onion, carrot and celery for about 5 minutes.
2. Add the garlic, jalapeño pepper, thyme and spices and sauté for about 1 minute.
3. Add the tomato paste, lentils and broth and bring to a boil.
4. Now, reduce the heat to low and simmer for about 2 hours.
5. Stir in the spinach and simmer for about 3-5 minutes.
6. Stir in cilantro and remove from the heat.

7. Serve hot.

8. Meal Prep Tip: Transfer the chili into a large bowl and set aside to cool. Divide the chili into 8 containers evenly. Cover the containers and refrigerate for 1-2 days. Reheat in the microwave before serving.

Nutrition Info: Calories 259 Total Fat 2.3 g Saturated Fat 0.3 g Cholesterol 0 mg Total Carbs 41 g Sugar 3.6 g Fiber 19 g Sodium 118 mg Potassium 856 mg Protein 18.2 g

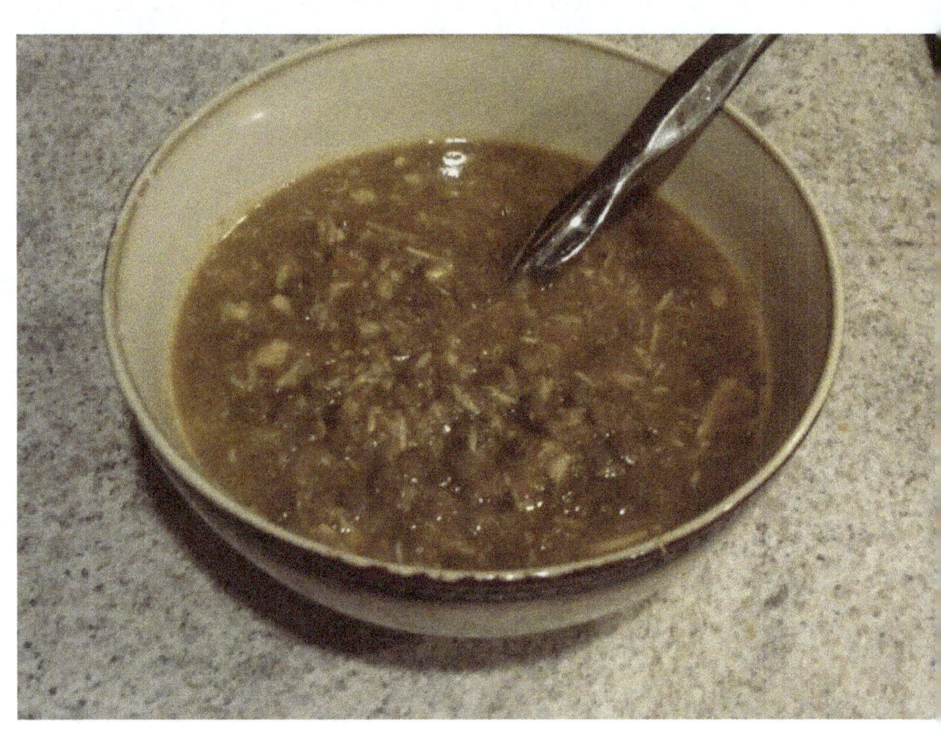

Fried Tofu Hotpot

Servings: 2

Cooking Time: 15 Minutes

Ingredients:

- 0.5lb fried tofu
- 1lb chopped Chinese vegetable mix
- 1 cup low sodium vegetable broth
- 2tbsp 5 spice seasoning
- 1tbsp smoked paprika

Directions:

1. Mix all the ingredients in your Instant Pot.
2. Cook on Stew for 15 minutes.
3. Release the pressure naturally.

Nutrition Info: Calories: 320 Carbs: 11 Sugar: 3 Fat: 23 Protein: 47 GL: 6

Seitan Curry

Servings: 2

Cooking Time: 20 Minutes

Ingredients:

- 0.5lb seitan
- 1 thinly sliced onion
- 1 cup chopped tomato
- 3tbsp curry paste
- 1tbsp oil or ghee

Directions:

1. Set the Instant Pot to saute and add the onion, oil, and curry paste.
2. When the onion is soft, add the remaining ingredients and seal.
3. Cook on Stew for 20 minutes.
4. Release the pressure naturally.

Nutrition Info: Calories: 240 Carbs: 19 Sugar: 4 Fat: 10 Protein: 32 GL: 10

Split Pea Stew

Servings: 2

Cooking Time: 35 Minutes

Ingredients:

- 1 cup dry split peas
- 1lb chopped vegetables
- 1 cup mushroom soup
- 2tbsp old bay seasoning

Directions:

1. Mix all the ingredients in your Instant Pot.
2. Cook on Beans for 35 minutes.
3. Release the pressure naturally.

Nutrition Info: Calories: 300 Carbs: 7 Sugar: 3 Fat: 2 Protein: 24 GL: 4

Grilled Potatoes In A Packet

Servings: 6

Cooking Time: 35 Minutes

Ingredients:

- 1 ½ lb. potatoes, sliced into wedges
- 2 cloves garlic, sliced
- 2 tablespoons olive oil
- Salt and pepper to taste
- 1 teaspoon dried rosemary

Directions:

1. Preheat your grill.
2. Create a packet using foil.
3. Drizzle oil over the potatoes and season with salt, pepper and rosemary.
4. Place potatoes inside the packet.
5. Fold and seal.
6. Grill for 15 minutes.
7. Turn to the other side.

8. Grill for 20 minutes.

9. Remove from the grill and open
    cautiously.

10. Serve while warm.

Nutrition Info: Calories 148 Total Fat 6 g Saturated Fat 1 g Cholesterol 0 mg Sodium 141 mg Total Carbohydrate 22 g Dietary Fiber 2 g Total Sugars 2 g Protein 3 g Potassium 626 mg

Seitan Roast

Servings: 2

Cooking Time: 35 Minutes

Ingredients:

- 1lb seitan roulade
- 1lb chopped winter vegetables
- 1 cup low sodium vegetable broth
- 4tbsp roast rub

Directions:

1. Rub the roast rub into your roulade.
2. Place the roulade and vegetables in your Instant Pot.
3. Add the broth. Seal.
4. Cook on Stew for 35 minutes.
5. Release the pressure naturally.

Nutrition Info: Calories: 260 Carbs: 9 Sugar: 2 Fat: 2 Protein: 49 GL: 4

Eggplant Curry

Servings: 2

Cooking Time: 20 Minutes

Ingredients:

- 2-3 cups chopped eggplant
- 1 thinly sliced onion
- 1 cup coconut milk
- 3tbsp curry paste
- 1tbsp oil or ghee

Directions:

1. Set the Instant Pot to saute and add the onion, oil, and curry paste.
2. When the onion is soft, add the remaining ingredients and seal.
3. Cook on Stew for 20 minutes.
4. Release the pressure naturally.

Nutrition Info: Calories: 350 Carbs: 15 Sugar: 3 Fat: 25 Protein: 11 GL: 10

Irish Stew

Servings: 2

Cooking Time: 35 Minutes

Ingredients:

- 1.5lb diced lamb shoulder
- 1lb chopped vegetables
- 1 cup low sodium beef broth
- 3 minced onions
- 1tbsp ghee

Directions:

1. Mix all the ingredients in your Instant Pot.
2. Cook on Stew for 35 minutes.
3. Release the pressure naturally.

Nutrition Info: Calories: 330; Carbs: 9; Sugar: 2; Fat: 12; Protein: 49; GL: 3

Vegetarian Split Pea Soup In A Crock Pot

Servings: 8

Cooking Time: 10 Minutes

Ingredients:

- 2 chopped ribs celery
- 2 cubes low-sodium bouillon
- 8 c. water
- 2 c. uncooked green split peas
- 3 bay leaves
- 2 carrots
- 2 chopped potatoes
- Pepper and salt

Directions:

1. In your Crock-Pot, put the bouillon cubes, split peas, and water. Stir a bit to break up the bouillon cubes.

2. Next, add the chopped potatoes, celery, and carrots followed with bay leaves.

3. Stir to combine well.

4. Cover and cook for at least 4 hours on your Crock-Pot's low setting or until the green split peas are soft.

5. Add a bit salt and pepper as needed.

6. Before serving, remove the bay leaves and enjoy.

Nutrition Info: Calories: 149, Fat:1 g, Carbs:30 g, Protein:7 g, Sugars:3 g, Sodium:732 mg

Thai Peanut, Carrot, & Shrimp Soup

Servings: 4

Cooking Time: 10 Minutes

Ingredients:

- 3 garlic cloves, minced
- ½ onion, sliced
- 1 tablespoon Thai red curry paste
- 1 tablespoon coconut oil
- fresh cilantro, minced, for garnish
- ½ pound shrimp, peeled and deveined
- ½ cup unsweetened plain almond milk
- 4 cups of low-sodium vegetable broth
- ½ cup whole unsalted peanuts
- 2 cups carrots, chopped

Directions:

1. In a pan, heat your oil over medium-high heat until shimmering.

2. Add your curry paste to the pan and cook continually stirring for about 1 minute. Add the garlic, onion, and carrots, along with peanuts to the pan. Continue cooking for 3 minutes or until your onion begins to soften.

3. Add your broth and bring to a boil. Reduce heat to a low setting and simmer for 6 minutes or until carrots are tender.

4. Use your immersion blender to puree your soup until smooth and return to pot. With heat setting on low, add the almond milk and stir to combine. Add your shrimp to the pot and cook for 3 minutes or until cooked.

5. Garnish soup with cilantro, then serve and enjoy!

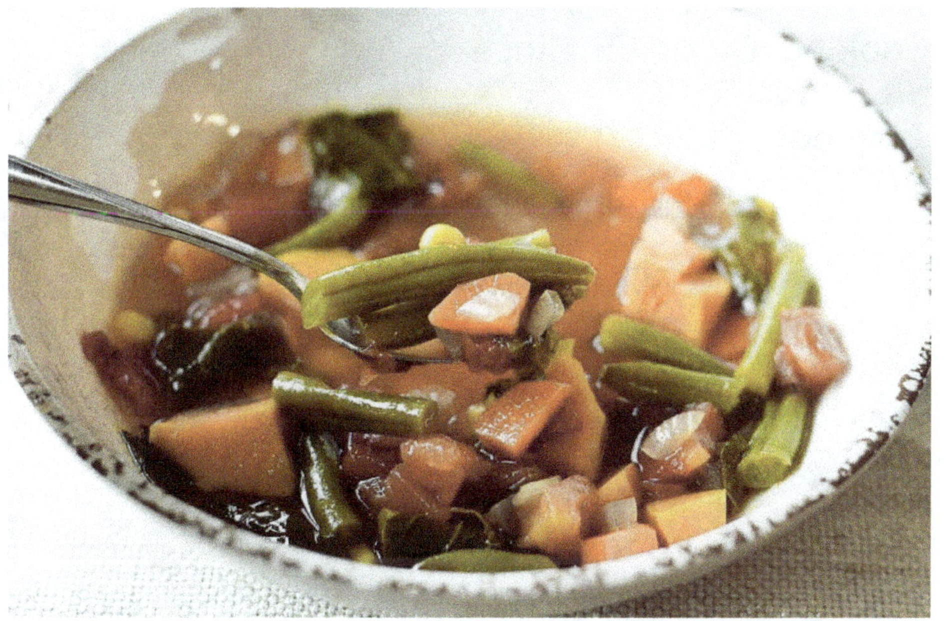

Ham Asparagus Soup

Servings: 3-4

Cooking Time: 55 Min.

Ingredients:

- 5 crushed garlic cloves
- 1 cup chopped ham
- 4 cups (preferably homemade) chicken broth
- 2 pounds trimmed and halved asparagus spears
- 2 tablespoons butter
- 1 chopped yellow onion
- ½ teaspoon dried thyme
- Salt and freshly (finely ground) black pepper, as per taste preference

Directions:

1. Arrange Instant Pot over a dry platform in your kitchen. Open its top lid and switch it on.

2. Find and press "SAUTE" cooking function; add the butter in it and allow it to heat.

3. In the pot, add the onions; cook (while stirring) until turns translucent and softened for around 4-5 minutes.

4. Add the garlic, ham bone and broth; stir, and cook for about 2-3 minutes.

5. Add the other ingredients; gently stir to mix well.

6. Close the lid to create a locked chamber; make sure that safety valve is in locking position.

7. Find and press "SOUP" cooking function; timer to 45 minutes with default "HIGH" pressure mode.

8. Allow the pressure to build to cook the ingredients.

9. After cooking time is over press "CANCEL" setting. Find and press "QPR" cooking function. This setting is for quick release of inside pressure.

10. Slowly open the lid, add the mix in a blender or processor.

11. Blend or process to make a smooth mix. Place the mix in serving bowls and enjoy the keto.

Nutrition Info: Calories - 146 Fat: 7g Saturated Fat: 3g Trans Fat: 0g Carbohydrates: 5g Fiber: 4g Sodium: 262mg Protein: 10g

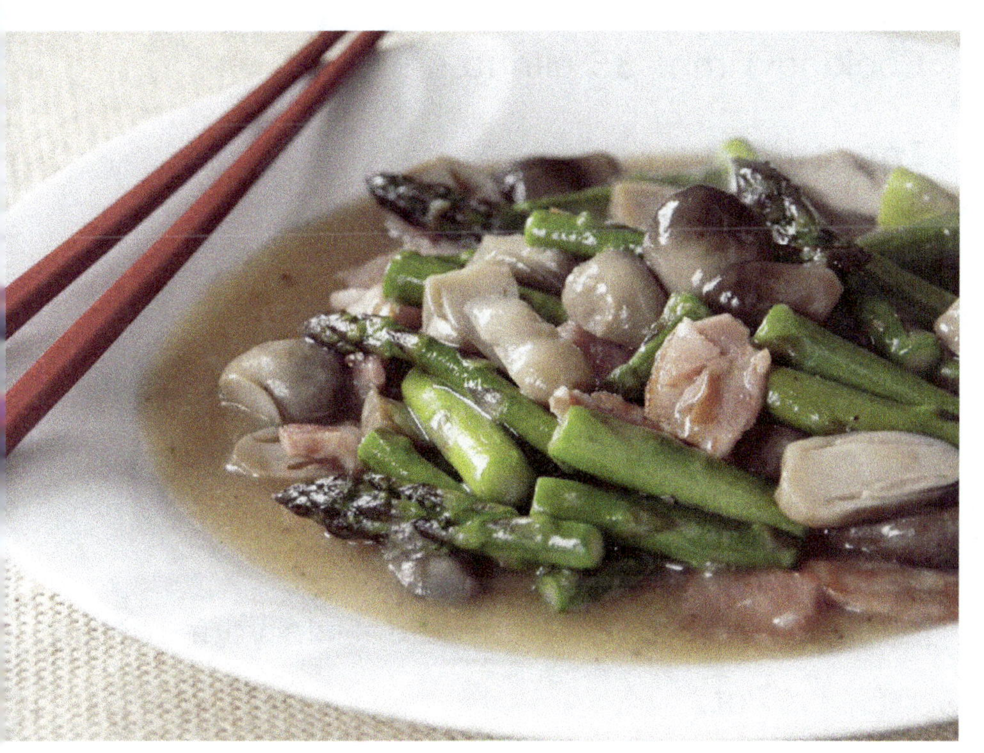

Cabbage Soup

Servings: 2

Cooking Time: 35 Minutes

Ingredients:

- 1lb shredded cabbage
- 1 cup low sodium vegetable broth
- 1 shredded onion
- 2tbsp mixed herbs
- 1tbsp black pepper

Directions:

1. Mix all the ingredients in your Instant Pot.
2. Cook on Stew for 35 minutes.
3. Release the pressure naturally.

Nutrition Info: Calories: 60; Carbs: 2; Sugar: 0; Fat: 2; Protein: 4; GL: 1

Chickpea Soup

Servings: 2

Cooking Time: 35 Minutes

Ingredients:

- 1lb cooked chickpeas
- 1lb chopped vegetables
- 1 cup low sodium vegetable broth
- 2tbsp mixed herbs

Directions:

1. Mix all the ingredients in your Instant Pot.
2. Cook on Stew for 35 minutes.
3. Release the pressure naturally.

Nutrition Info: Calories: 310; Carbs: 20; Sugar: 3; Fat: 5; Protein: 27; GL: 5

Meatball Stew

Servings: 2

Cooking Time: 25 Minutes

Ingredients:

- 1lb sausage meat
- 2 cups chopped tomato
- 1 cup chopped vegetables
- 2tbsp Italian seasonings
- 1tbsp vegetable oil

Directions:

1. Roll the sausage into meatballs.
2. Put the Instant Pot on Sauté and fry the meatballs in the oil until brown.
3. Mix all the ingredients in your Instant Pot.
4. Cook on Stew for 25 minutes.
5. Release the pressure naturally.

Nutrition Info: Calories: 300; Carbs: 4; Sugar: 1; Fat: 12; Protein: 40; GL: 2

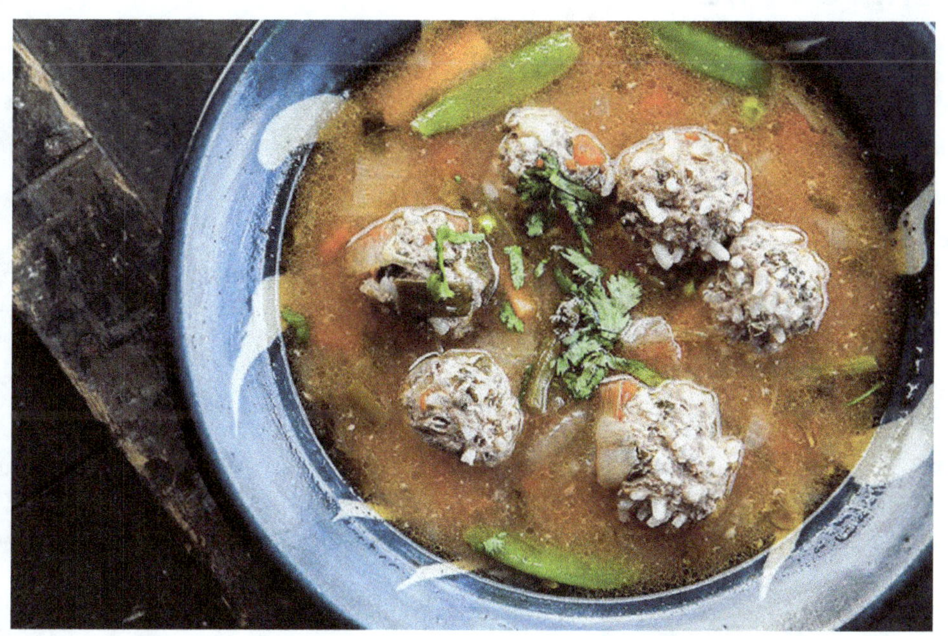

Squash Soup

Servings: 6

Cooking Time: 8 Hours

Ingredients:

- 2 lb butternut squash, peeled, chopped into chunks
- 1 tsp ginger, minced
- 1/4 tsp cinnamon
- 1 Tbsp curry powder
- 2 bay leaves
- 1 tsp black pepper
- 1/2 cup heavy cream
- 2 cups chicken stock
- 1 Tbsp garlic, minced
- 2 carrots, cut into chunks
- 2 apples, peeled, cored and diced
- 1 large onion, diced
- 1 tsp salt

Directions:

1. Spray a crock pot inside with cooking spray.
2. Add all ingredients except cream to the crock pot and stir well.
3. Cover and cook on low for 8 hours.
4. Purée the soup using an immersion blender until smooth and creamy.
5. Stir in heavy cream and season soup with pepper and salt.
6. Serve and enjoy.

Nutrition Info: Calories 170 Fat 4.4 g Carbohydrates 34.4 g Sugar 13.4g Protein 2.9 g Cholesterol 14 mg

French Onion Soup

Servings: 2

Cooking Time: 35 Minutes

Ingredients:

- 6 onions, chopped finely
- 2 cups vegetable broth
- 2tbsp oil
- 2tbsp Gruyere

Directions:

1. Place the oil in your Instant Pot and cook the onions on Sauté until soft and brown.
2. Mix all the ingredients in your Instant Pot.
3. Cook on Stew for 35 minutes.
4. Release the pressure naturally.

Nutrition Info: Calories: 110; Carbs: 8; Sugar: 3; Fat: 10; Protein: 3; GL: 4

Cherry Stew

Servings: 6

Cooking Time: 10 Minutes

Ingredients:

- 2 c. water
- ½ c. powered cocoa
- ¼ c. coconut sugar
- 1 lb. pitted cherries

Directions:

1. In a pan, combine the cherries with all the water, sugar plus the hot chocolate mix, stir, cook over medium heat for ten minutes, divide into bowls and serve cold.
2. Enjoy!

Nutrition Info: Calories: 207, Fat:1 g, Carbs:8 g, Protein:6 g, Sugars:27 g, Sodium:19 mg

Curried Carrot Soup

Servings: 6

Cooking Time: 5 Minutes

Ingredients:

- 2 celery stalks, chopped
- 1 small onion, chopped
- 1 tablespoon extra-virgin olive oil
- 1 tablespoon fresh cilantro, chopped
- ¼ teaspoon freshly ground black pepper
- 1 cup of canned coconut milk
- ¼ teaspoon salt
- 4 cups of low-sodium vegetable broth
- 6 medium carrots, roughly chopped
- 1 teaspoon fresh ginger, minced
- 1 teaspoon ground cumin
- 1 ½ teaspoon curry powder

Directions:

1.   Heat your Instant Pot to high setting and add the olive oil.

2.   Sauté your celery and onion for 3 minutes. Add the curry powder, ginger, and cumin to the pot and cook for about 30 seconds.

3.   Add the carrots, vegetable broth, and salt to your pot. Close pot and seal and set on high for 5 minutes. Allow the pressure to release naturally.

4.   Pure your soup in batches in a blender jar and transfer back into the pot.

5.   Stir in the coconut milk along with pepper and heat through. Top soup with cilantro, then serve and enjoy!

Nutrition Info: Carbs per serving: 13g

Vegan Cream Soup With Avocado & Zucchini

Servings: 2

Cooking Time: 20 Minutes

Ingredients:

- 3 tsp vegetable oil
- 1 leek, chopped
- 1 rutabaga, sliced
- 3 cups zucchinis, chopped
- 1 avocado, chopped
- Salt and black pepper to taste
- 4 cups vegetable broth
- 2 tbsp fresh mint, chopped

Directions:

1. In a pot, sauté leek, zucchini, and rutabaga in warm oil for about 7-10 minutes. Season with black pepper and salt. Pour in broth and bring to a boil.

Lower the heat and simmer for 20 minutes.

2. Lift from the heat. In batches, add the soup and avocado to a blender. Blend until creamy and smooth. Serve in bowls topped with fresh mint.

Nutrition Info: Calories 378 Fat: 24.5g, Net Carbs: 9.3g, Protein: 8.2g

Kebab Stew

Servings: 2

Cooking Time: 35 Minutes

Ingredients:

- 1lb cubed, seasoned kebab meat
- 1lb cooked chickpeas
- 1 cup low sodium vegetable broth
- 1tbsp black pepper

Directions:

1. Mix all the ingredients in your Instant Pot.
2. Cook on Stew for 35 minutes.
3. Release the pressure naturally.

Nutrition Info: Calories: 290; Carbs: 22; Sugar: 4; Fat: 10; Protein: 34; GL: 6

Meatless Ball Soup

Servings: 2

Cooking Time: 15 Minutes

Ingredients:

- 1lb minced tofu
- 0.5lb chopped vegetables
- 2 cups low sodium vegetable broth
- 1tbsp almond flour
- salt and pepper

Directions:

1. Mix the tofu, flour, salt and pepper.
2. Form the meatballs.
3. Place all the ingredients in your Instant Pot.
4. Cook on Stew for 15 minutes.
5. Release the pressure naturally.

Nutrition Info: Calories: 240; Carbs: 9; Sugar: 3; Fat: 10; Protein: 35; GL: 5

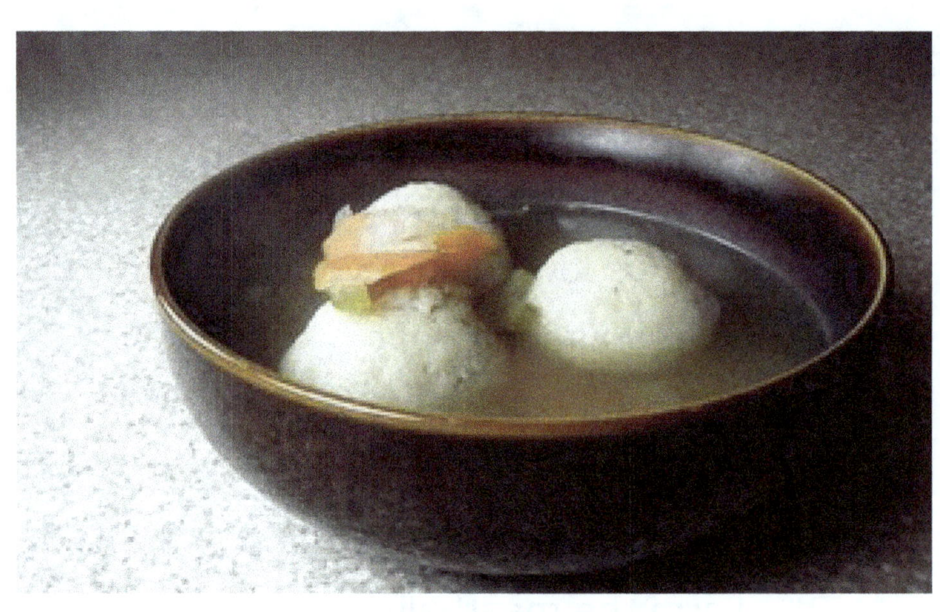

Tofu Soup

Servings: 8

Cooking Time: 10 Minutes

Ingredients:

- 1 lb. cubed extra-firm tofu
- 3 diced medium carrots
- 8 c. low-sodium vegetable broth
- ½ tsp. freshly ground white pepper
- 8 minced garlic cloves
- 6 sliced and divided scallions
- 4 oz. sliced mushrooms
- 1-inch minced fresh ginger piece

Directions:

1. Pour the broth into a stockpot. Add all of the ingredients except for the tofu and last 2 scallions. Bring to a boil over high heat.

2.   Once boiling, add the tofu. Reduce heat to low, cover, and simmer for 5 minutes.

3.   Remove from heat, ladle soup into bowls, and garnish with the remaining sliced scallions. Serve immediately.

Nutrition Info: Calories: 91, Fat:3 g, Carbs:8 g, Protein:6 g, Sugars:4 g, Sodium:900 mg

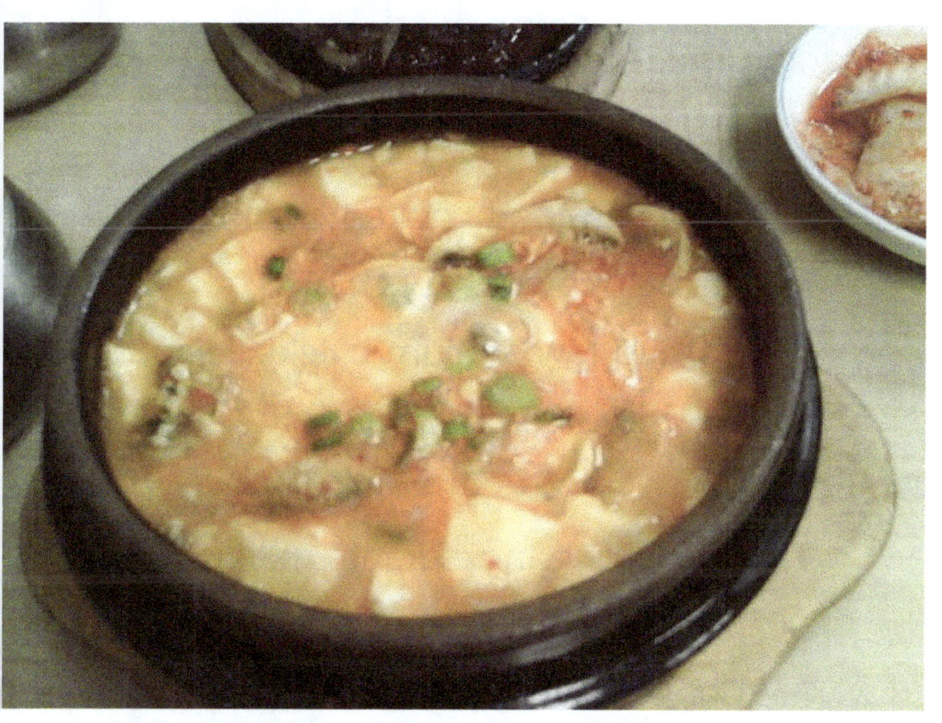

Chicken Zoodle Soup

Servings: 2

Cooking Time: 35 Minutes

Ingredients:

- 1lb chopped cooked chicken
- 1lb spiralized zucchini
- 1 cup low sodium chicken soup
- 1 cup diced vegetables

Directions:

1. Mix all the ingredients except the zucchini in your Instant Pot.
2. Cook on Stew for 35 minutes.
3. Release the pressure naturally.
4. Stir in the zucchini and allow to heat thoroughly.

Nutrition Info: Calories: 250; Carbs: 5; Sugar: 0; Fat: 10; Protein: 40; GL: 1

Cheese Cream Soup With Chicken & Cilantro

Servings: 4

Cooking Time: 10 Minutes

Ingredients:

- 1 carrot, chopped
- 1 onion, chopped
- 2 cups cooked and shredded chicken
- 3 tbsp butter
- 4 cups chicken broth
- 2 tbsp cilantro, chopped
- 1/3 cup buffalo sauce
- ½ cup cream cheese
- Salt and black pepper, to taste

Directions:

1. In a skillet over medium heat, warm butter and sauté carrot and onion until tender, about 5 minutes.

2. Add to a food processor and blend with buffalo sauce and cream cheese, until smooth. Transfer to a pot, add chicken broth and heat until hot but do not bring to a boil. Stir in chicken, salt, pepper and cook until heated through. When ready, remove to soup bowls and serve garnished with cilantro.

Nutrition Info: Calories 487, Fat: 41g, Net Carbs: 7.2g, Protein: 16.3g

Spicy Pepper Soup

Servings: 2

Cooking Time: 15 Minutes

Ingredients:

- 1lb chopped mixed sweet peppers
- 1 cup low sodium vegetable broth
- 3tbsp chopped chili peppers
- 1tbsp black pepper

Directions:

1. Mix all the ingredients in your Instant Pot.
2. Cook on Stew for 15 minutes.
3. Release the pressure naturally. Blend.

Nutrition Info: Calories: 100; Carbs: 11; Sugar: 4; Fat: 2; Protein: 3; GL: 6

Awesome Chicken Enchilada Soup

Servings: 4

Cooking Time: 30 Minutes

Ingredients:

- 2 tbsp coconut oil
- 1 lb boneless, skinless chicken thighs
- ¾ cup red enchilada sauce, sugar-free
- ¼ cup water
- ¼ cup onion, chopped
- 3 oz canned diced green chilis
- 1 avocado, sliced
- 1 cup cheddar cheese, shredded
- ¼ cup pickled jalapeños, chopped
- ½ cup sour cream
- 1 tomato, diced

Directions:

1. Put a large pan over medium heat. Add coconut oil and warm. Place in the chicken and cook until browned on the outside. Stir in onion, chillis, water, and enchilada sauce, then close with a lid.
2. Allow simmering for 20 minutes until the chicken is cooked through.
3. Spoon the soup on a serving bowl and top with the sauce, cheese, sour cream, tomato, and avocado.

Nutrition Info: Calories: 643, Fat: 44.2g, Net Carbs: 9.7g, Protein: 45.8g

Zucchini-basil Soup

Servings: 5

Cooking Time: 10 Minutes

Ingredients:

- 1/3 c. packed basil leaves
- ¾ c. chopped onion
- ¼ c. olive oil
- 2 lbs. trimmed and sliced zucchini
- 2 chopped garlic cloves
- 4 c. divided water

Directions:

1. Peel and julienne the skin from half of zucchini; toss with 1/2 teaspoon salt and drain in a sieve until wilted, at least 20 minutes. Coarsely chop remaining zucchini.

2. Cook onion and garlic in oil in a saucepan over medium-low heat,

stirring occasionally, until onions are translucent. Add chopped zucchini and 1 teaspoon salt and cook, stirring occasionally.

3. Add 3 cups water and simmer with the lid ajar until tender. Pour the soup in a blender and purée soup with basil.

4. Bring remaining cup water to a boil in a small saucepan and blanch julienned zucchini. Drain.

5. Top soup with julienned zucchini. Season soup with salt and pepper and serve.

Nutrition Info: Calories: 169.3, Fat:13.7 g, Carbs:12 g, Protein:2 g,Sugars:3.8 g, Sodium:8 mg

Sweet And Sour Soup

Servings: 2

Cooking Time: 35 Minutes

Ingredients:

- 1lb cubed chicken breast
- 1lb chopped vegetables
- 1 cup low carb sweet and sour sauce
- 0.5 cup diabetic marmalade

Directions:

1. Mix all the ingredients in your Instant Pot.
2. Cook on Stew for 35 minutes.
3. Release the pressure naturally.

Nutrition Info: Calories: 305; Carbs: 4; Sugar: 1.2; Fat: 12; Protein: 40; GL: 2

Curried Shrimp & Green Bean Soup

Servings: 4

Cooking Time: 10 Minutes

Ingredients:

- 1 onion, chopped
- 2 tbsp red curry paste
- 2 tbsp butter
- 1-pound jumbo shrimp, peeled and deveined
- 2 tsp ginger-garlic puree
- 1 cup coconut milk
- Salt and chili pepper to taste
- 1 bunch green beans, halved
- 1 tbsp cilantro, chopped

Directions:

1. Add the shrimp to melted butter in a saucepan over medium heat, season with salt and pepper, and cook until they are opaque, 2 to 3 minutes. Remove to a plate. Add in the ginger-garlic puree, onion, and red curry paste and sauté for 2 minutes until fragrant.

2. Stir in the coconut milk; add the shrimp, salt, chili pepper, and green beans. Cook for 4 minutes. Reduce the heat to a simmer and cook an additional 3 minutes, occasionally stirring. Adjust taste with salt, fetch soup into serving bowls, and serve sprinkled with cilantro.

Nutrition Info: Calories 351, Fat 32.4g, Net Carbs 3.2g, Protein 7.7g

Beef Borscht Soup

Servings: 8

Cooking Time: 30 Minutes

Ingredients:

- 2 lbs ground beef
- 3 beets, peeled and diced
- 2 large carrots, diced
- 3 stalks of celery, diced
- 1 onion, diced
- 2 cloves garlic, diced
- 3 cups shredded cabbage
- 6 cups beef stock
- ½ tbsp thyme
- 1 bay leaf
- Salt and ground black pepper to taste

Directions:

1. Preheat the Instant Pot by selecting SAUTÉ.

2. Add the ground beef and cook, stirring, for 5 minutes, until browned.

3. Combine all the rest ingredients in the Instant Pot and stir to mix. Close and lock the lid.

4. Press the CANCEL button to stop the SAUTE function, then select the MANUAL setting and set the cooking time for 15 minutes at HIGH pressure.

5. Once timer goes off, allow to Naturally Release for 10 minutes, then release any remaining pressure manually. Uncover the pot.

6. Let the dish sit for 5-10 minutes and serve.

Nutrition Info: Calories 301 Fat 27.2 g Carbohydrates 13.6 g Sugar 6 g Protein 3 g Cholesterol 33 mg

Broccoli & Spinach Soup

Servings: 4

Cooking Time: 20 Minutes

Ingredients:

- 2 tbsp butter
- 1 onion, chopped
- 1 garlic clove, minced
- 2 heads broccoli, cut in florets
- 2 stalks celery, chopped
- 4 cups vegetable broth
- 1 cup baby spinach
- Salt and black pepper to taste
- 1 tbsp basil, chopped
- Parmesan cheese, shaved to serve

Directions:

1. Melt the butter in a saucepan over medium heat. Sauté the garlic and onion for 3 minutes until softened. Mix

in the broccoli and celery, and cook for 4 minutes until slightly tender. Pour in the broth, bring to a boil, then reduce the heat to medium-low and simmer covered for about 5 minutes.

2. Drop in the spinach to wilt, adjust the seasonings, and cook for 4 minutes. Ladle soup into serving bowls. Serve with a sprinkle of grated Parmesan cheese and chopped basil.

Nutrition Info: Calories 123 Fat 11g Net Carbs 3.2g Protein 1.8g

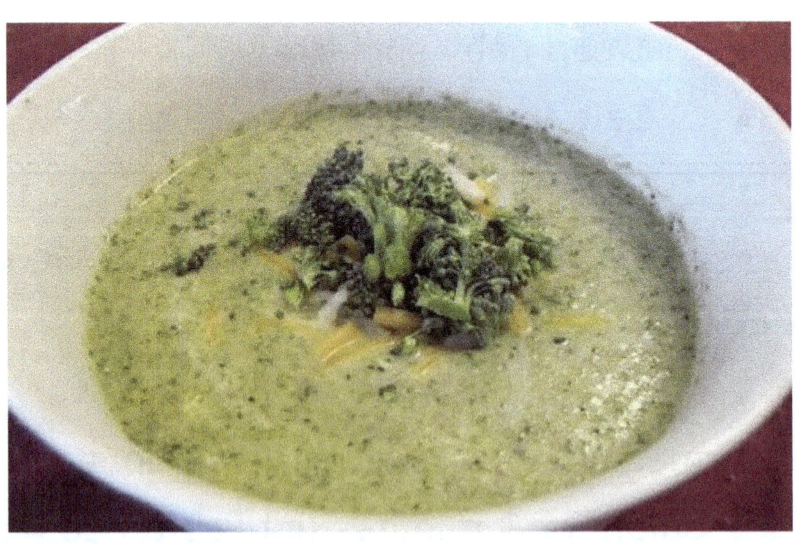

Vegetable Chicken Soup

Servings: 6

Cooking Time: 6 Hours

Ingredients:

- 4 cups chicken, boneless, skinless, cooked and diced
- 4 tsp garlic, minced
- 2/3 cups onion, diced
- 1 1/2 cups carrot, diced
- 6 cups chicken stock
- 2 Tbsp lime juice
- 1/4 cup jalapeño pepper, diced
- 1/2 cup tomatoes, diced
- 1/2 cup fresh cilantro, chopped
- 1 tsp chili powder
- 1 Tbsp cumin
- 1 3/4 cups tomato juice
- 2 tsp sea salt

Directions:

1. Add all ingredients to a crock pot and stir well.
2. Cover and cook on low for 6 hours.
3. Stir well and serve.

Nutrition Info: Calories 192 Fat 3.8 g Carbohydrates 9.8 g Sugar 5.7 g Protein 29.2 g Cholesterol 72 mg

Beef Barley Soup

Servings: 8

Cooking Time: 30 Minutes

Ingredients:

- 2 tbsp olive oil
- 2 lbs beef chuck roast, cut into 1½ inch steaks
- Salt and ground black pepper to taste
- 2 onions, chopped
- 4 cloves of garlic, sliced
- 4 large carrots, chopped
- 1 stalk of celery, chopped
- 1 cup pearl barley, rinsed
- 1 bay leaf
- 8 cups chicken stock
- 1 tbsp fish sauce

Directions:

1. Select the SAUTÉ setting on the Instant Pot and heat the oil.
2. Sprinkle the beef with salt and pepper. Put in the pot and brown for about 5 minutes. Turn and brown the other side.
3. Remove the meat from the pot.
4. Add the onion, garlic, carrots, and celery. Stir and sauté for 6 minutes.
5. Return the beef to the pot. Add the pearl barley, bay leaf, chicken stock and fish sauce. Stir well.
6. Close and lock the lid. Press the CANCEL button to reset the cooking program, then press the MANUAL button and set the cooking time for 30 minutes at HIGH pressure.
7. Once cooking is complete, let the pressure Release Naturally for 15

minutes. Release any remaining steam manually. Uncover the pot.

8. Remove cloves garlic, large vegetable chunks and bay leaf.

9. Taste for seasoning and add more salt if needed.

Nutrition Info: Calories 200 Fat 27.2 g Carbohydrates 13.6 g Sugar 2 g Protein 4.4 g Cholesterol 32 mg

Sirloin Carrot Soup

Servings: 6

Cooking Time: 10 Minutes

Ingredients:

- 1 lb. chopped carrots and celery mix
- 32 oz. low-sodium beef stock
- 1/3 c. whole-wheat flour
- 1 lb. ground beef sirloin
- 1 tbsp. olive oil
- 1 chopped yellow onion

Directions:

1. Heat up the olive oil in a saucepan over medium-high flame; add the beef and the flour.
2. Stir well and cook to brown for 4-5 minutes.
3. Add the celery, onion, carrots, and stock; stir and bring to a simmer.

4. Turn down the heat to low and cook
    for 12-15 minutes.

5. Serve warm.

Nutrition Info: Calories: 140, Fat: 4.5 g,Carbs: 16 g, Protein: 9 g, Sugars: 3 g, Sodium:670 mg

Mexican Chicken Soup

Servings: 6

Cooking Time: 4 Hours

Ingredients:

- 1 1/2 lb chicken thighs, skinless and boneless
- 14 oz chicken stock
- 14 oz salsa
- 8 oz Monterey Jack cheese, shredded

Directions:

1. Place chicken into a crock pot.
2. Pour remaining ingredients over the chicken.
3. Cover and cook on high for 4 hours.
4. Remove chicken from crock pot and shred using forks.
5. Return shredded chicken to the crock pot and stir well.

6. Serve and enjoy.

Nutrition Info: Calories 371 Fat 19.5 g Carbohydrates 5.7 g Sugar 2.2 g Protein 42.1 g Cholesterol 135 mg

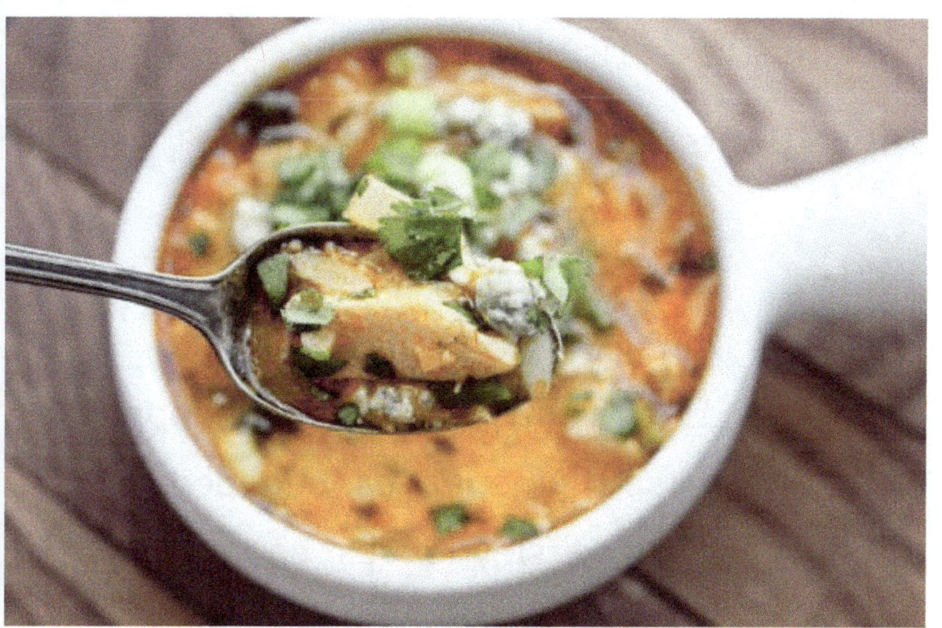

Mushroom Cream Soup With Herbs

Servings: 4

Cooking Time: 15 Minutes

Ingredients:

- 1 onion, chopped
- ½ cup crème fraiche
- ¼ cup butter
- 12 oz white mushrooms, chopped
- 1 tsp thyme leaves, chopped
- 1 tsp parsley leaves, chopped
- 1 tsp cilantro leaves, chopped
- 2 garlic cloves, minced
- 4 cups vegetable broth
- Salt and black pepper, to taste

Directions:

1. Add butter, onion and garlic to a large pot over high heat and cook for 3

minutes until tender. Add mushrooms, salt and pepper, and cook for 10 minutes. Pour in the broth and bring to a boil.

2. Reduce the heat and simmer for 10 minutes. Puree the soup with a hand blender until smooth. Stir in crème fraiche. Garnish with herbs before serving.

Nutrition Info: Calories 213 Fat: 18g Net Carbs: 4.1g Protein: 3.1g

Beef & Mushroom Barley Soup

Servings: 6

Cooking Time: 1 Hour And 20 Minutes

Ingredients:

- ½ cup of pearl barley
- 1 cup of water
- 4 cups of low-sodium beef broth
- ½ teaspoon thyme, dried
- 6 garlic cloves, minced
- 3 celery stalks, chopped
- 1 onion, chopped
- 2 carrots, chopped
- 8-ounces of mushrooms, sliced
- 1 tablespoon extra-virgin olive oil
- ¼ teaspoon freshly ground black pepper
- 1 lb. Of beef stew meat, cubed

Directions:

1. Season your meat with salt and pepper.

2.   Heat the oil in an Instant Pot over high heat. Add the beef and brown, then remove meat and set aside.

3. Add your mushrooms to the pot and cook for about 1 to 2 minutes or until they begin to soften. Remove the mushrooms from pot and set them aside along with the meat.

4. Add your carrots, celery, and onions into the pot. Sauté vegetables for about 4 minutes or until they begin to soften. Add your garlic into pot and cook until fragrant.

5. Place the meat and mushrooms back into the pot, then add the beef broth, thyme, and water. Set your pot pressure to high and cook for 15

minutes. Allow the pressure to release naturally.

6. Open your Instant Pot and add the barley. Use the slow cooker function on the pot, with the lid having vent open, then continue cooking for an additional hour or until your barley is cooked and tender. Serve and enjoy!

Nutrition Info: Carbs per serving: 19g

Spicy Chicken Pepper Stew

Servings: 6

Cooking Time: 6 Hours

Ingredients:

- 3 chicken breasts, skinless and boneless, cut into small pieces
- 1 tsp garlic, minced
- 1 tsp ground ginger
- 2 tsp olive oil
- 2 tsp soy sauce
- 1 Tbsp fresh lemon juice
- 1/2 cup green onions, sliced
- 1 Tbsp crushed red pepper
- 8 oz chicken stock
- 1 bell pepper, chopped
- 1 green chili pepper, sliced
- 2 jalapeño peppers, sliced
- 1/2 tsp black pepper

- • 1/4 tsp sea salt

Directions:

1. Add all ingredients to a large mixing bowl and mix well. Place in the refrigerator overnight.
2. Pour marinated chicken mixture into a crock pot.
3. Cover and cook on low for 6 hours.
4. Stir well and serve.

Nutrition Info: Calories 171 Fat 7.4 g Carbohydrates 3.7 g Sugar 1.7 g Protein 22 g Cholesterol 65 mg

Cream Pepper Stew

Servings: 4

Cooking Time: 10 Min.

Ingredients:

- 1 (preferably medium size) celery stalk, chopped
- 1 (preferably medium size) yellow bell pepper, chopped
- 1 (preferably medium size) green bell pepper, chopped
- 2 large red bell peppers, chopped
- 1 small red onion, chopped
- 2 tablespoons butter
- 1/2 cup cream cheese, full-fat
- 1/4 teaspoon dried thyme, (finely ground)
- 1/2 teaspoon black pepper, (finely ground)

- 1 teaspoon dried parsley, (finely ground)
- 1 teaspoon salt
- 2 cups vegetable stock
- 1 cup heavy cream

Directions:

1. Arrange Instant Pot over a dry platform in your kitchen. Open its top lid and switch it on.

2. Find and press "SAUTE" cooking function; add the butter in it and allow it to heat.

3. In the pot, add the onions, bell pepper, and celery; cook (while stirring) until turns translucent and softened for around 3-4 minutes.

4. Pour in the vegetable stock and heavy cream — season with salt, pepper, parsley, and thyme.

5. Close the lid to create a locked chamber; make sure that safety valve is in locking position.

6. Find and press "MANUAL" cooking function; timer to 6 minutes with default "HIGH" pressure mode.

7. Allow the pressure to build to cook the ingredients.

8. After cooking time is over press "CANCEL" setting. Find and press "QPR" cooking function. This setting is for quick release of inside pressure.

9. Slowly open the lid, mix in the cream; take out the cooked in serving plates or serving bowls, and enjoy the keto .

Nutrition Info: Calories - 286 Fat: 27g Saturated Fat: 6g Trans Fat: 0g Carbohydrates: 9g Fiber: 3g Sodium: 523mg Protein: 5g

Easy Beef Mushroom Stew

Servings: 8

Cooking Time: 8 Hours

Ingredients:

- 2 lb stewing beef, cubed
- 1 packet dry onion soup mix
- 4 oz can mushrooms, sliced
- 14 oz can cream of mushroom soup
- 1/2 cup water
- 1/4 tsp black pepper
- 1/2 tsp salt

Directions:

1. Spray a crock pot inside with cooking spray.
2. Add all ingredients into the crock pot and stir well.
3. Cover and cook on low for 8 hours.
4. Stir well and serve.

Nutrition Info: Calories 237 Fat 8.5 g Carbohydrates 2.7 g Sugar 0.4 g Protein 35.1 g Cholesterol 101 mg

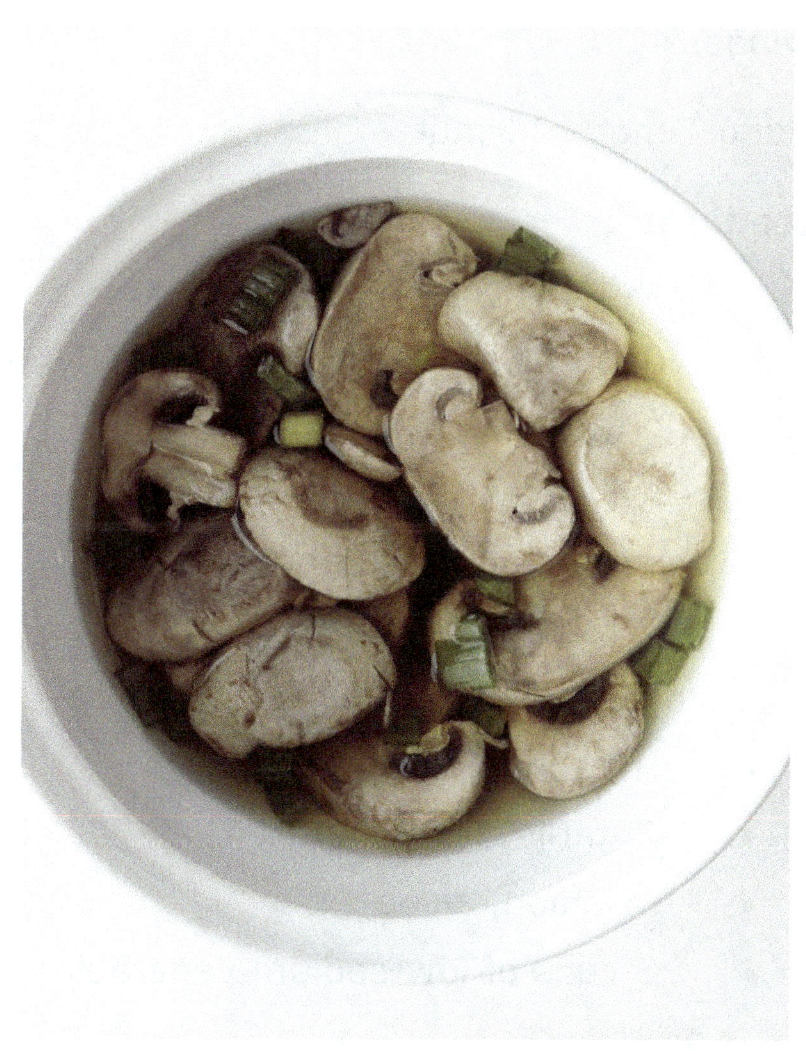

Summer Squash Soup With Crispy Chickpeas

Servings: 4

Cooking Time: 20 Minutes

Ingredients:

- ¼ teaspoon smoked paprika
- 1 teaspoon extra-virgin olive oil, plus one tablespoon
- 1 (15-ounce) can low-sodium chickpeas, drained and rinsed
- 2 tablespoons plain low-fat Greek yogurt
- freshly ground black pepper
- 3 garlic cloves, minced
- ½ onion, diced
- 3 cups of low-sodium vegetable broth

- 3 medium zucchinis, coarsely chopped

- pinch of sea salt, plus ½ teaspoon

Directions:

1. Preheat your oven to 425° Fahrenheit. Line a baking sheet with some parchment paper.

2. In a mixing bowl, toss your chickpeas with one teaspoon of olive oil, the smoked paprika, and a pinch of sea salt. Transfer your mixture to the baking sheet, then roast until crispy for about 20 minutes, stirring once. Set aside.

3. In a pot, heat the remaining 1 tablespoon of oil over medium heat.

4. Add your zucchini, onion, broth, and garlic to the pot and bring to a boil. Lower the heat to simmer, then cook until the onion and zucchini are tender, for about 20 minutes.

5. In a blender jar, puree your soup, then return it to the pot.

6. Add the yogurt, and the remaining ½ teaspoon of sea salt, and pepper, then stir well. Serve topped with roasted chickpeas and enjoy!

Nutrition Info: Carbs per serving: 24g

Healthy Chicken Kale Soup

Servings: 6

Cooking Time: 6 Hours 15 Minutes

Ingredients:

- 2 lb chicken breasts, skinless and boneless
- 1/4 cup fresh lemon juice
- 5 oz baby kale
- 32 oz chicken stock
- 1/2 cup olive oil
- 1 large onion, sliced
- 14 oz chicken broth
- 1 Tbsp extra-virgin olive oil
- Salt

Directions:

1. Heat the extra-virgin olive oil in a pan over medium heat.
2. Season chicken with salt and place in the hot pan.
3. Cover pan and cook chicken for 15 minutes.
4. Remove chicken from the pan and shred it using forks.
5. Add shredded chicken to a crock pot.
6. Add sliced onion, olive oil, and broth to a blender and blend until combined.
7. Pour blended mixture into the crock pot.
8. Add remaining ingredients to the crock pot and stir well.
9. Cover and cook on low for 6 hours.
10. Stir well and serve.

Nutrition Info: Calories 493 Fat 31.3 g Carbohydrates 5.8 g Sugar 1.9 g Protein 46.7 g Cholesterol 135 mg